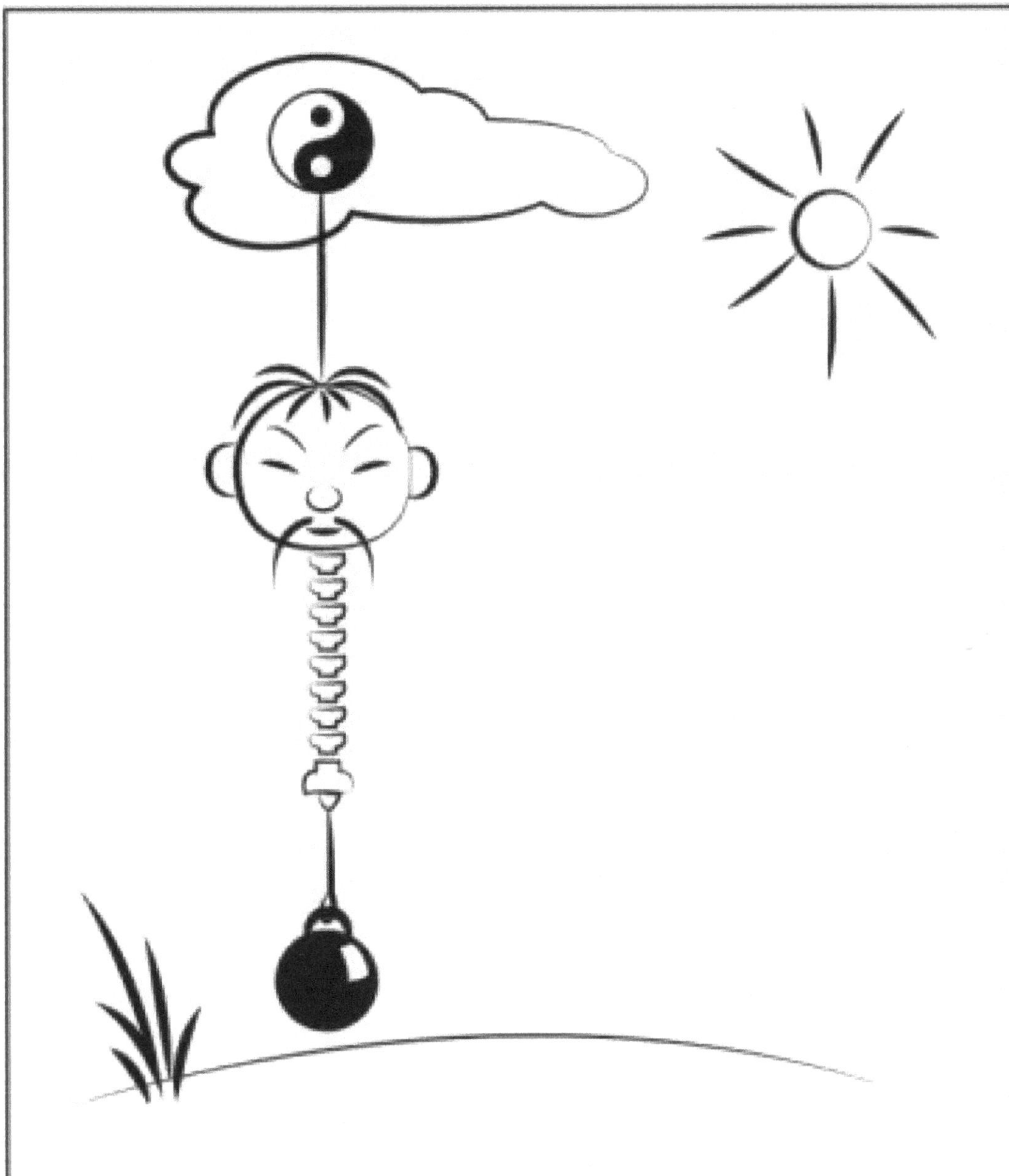

# ACCEPT THE FORCE OF GRAVITY

Qigong and Taichi benefits
My experience in China in simple words

ANDREA LAFFRANCHINI

EBOOK ISBN: 978-9-69-739209-4

PAPERBACK ISBN: 978-9-69-739210-0

HARDBACK ISBN: 978-9-69-739211-7

# Dedication

To Sara, my Sara.
Ti amo

To Coach Mike, a man of honesty and integrity, a great expert in sports performance, and a friend to have.
Thank you

To Dr. Alvydas, an extraordinary connoisseur of the human body who gives with love without asking.
Thank you

To Dr. Jyun, a humble and passionate enthusiast and expert in well-being.
Thank you

To Mario, a respectful and open-minded man, a great massage expert, and a loyal friend.
Thank you

# Contents

FOREWORD ..... 1
Sara Della Bruna ..... 1
Coach Mike Cunliffe ..... 3
Dr. Jyun Shimizu ..... 4
INTRODUCTION ..... 5
MY TRAVEL TO CHINA ..... 7
QI, OUR VITAL ENERGY ..... 12
The meridians ..... 12
Meridians in Qigong and Taichi ..... 13
REVERSE BREATHING ..... 15
MASSAGE TAPPING ..... 16
Soft hammer ..... 16
Cuppy palm ..... 16
Comb massage ..... 17
Hand massage ..... 18
MEDITATION ..... 19
What it is about ..... 19
How to do it ..... 21
WARM-UP EXERCISES ..... 24
Neck ..... 24
Shoulder ..... 24
Lower back ..... 25
Legs ..... 25

Two hands hold the feet to strengthen the kidneys and waist ........ 26

QIGONG ........ 27

Benefits of Qigong ........ 27

Qigong exercises ........ 28

Qigong benefits for each exercise ........ 33

More to know ........ 37

Summary Qigong Table ........ 38

TAICHI ........ 39

Characteristics of Taichi movements ........ 39

Benefits of Taichi ........ 40

Taichi exercises ........ 41

More to know ........ 48

Summary Taichi Table ........ 48

SIMILARITIES AND DIFFERENCES BETWEEN QIGONG AND TAICHI ........ 49

COMBAT ........ 51

DYNAMIC STRETCHING ........ 52

Stretch the lower back n.1 ........ 52

Stretch the lower back n.2 ........ 53

THE MOVEMENT BEHIND TAICHI ........ 55

One hand ........ 56

First circle ........ 56

Second circle ........ 57

Third circle ........ 57

Fourth circle ........ 58

Two hands ........ 59

Seventh circle ........ 59

Eighth circle ........ 60

Ninth and tenth circles ........ 61

THE FORCE OF GRAVITY ........ 62

THE PUPPET ........ 64

RUNNING AND MEDITATION ........ 65

ENERGYUPPROBIOTIC ........ 67

Red Korean Ginseng & Probiotics ........ 67

Gut health boost ........ 68

PRACTICE ........ 70

B&B CUORE ALPINO ........ 71

CONCLUSION ........ 72

ABOUT THE AUTHOR ........ 73

QIGONG & TAICHI CERTIFICATION ........ 74

# Foreword

## Sara Della Bruna

### Why Read This Book

Accept the Force of Gravity is a manual with the flavor of a novel. It is a book that can ignite curiosity, that surprises and, perhaps because it was written by Andrea, who had no previous knowledge of the subject, is extremely free of prejudice or pre-packaged points of view, and therefore delivers authentic pages linked to a deep personal experience.

It can be read by those who, like me, have no knowledge of Taichi or Qigong, as it introduces concepts that, although far removed from Western culture, somehow seem to be recognized and manage to 'speak' to a deep part of us that perhaps 'remembers'. Page after page, the desire to approach these disciplines whose movements seem like delicate but stable choreographies is born. It's a kind of dance suitable for everyone, which brings with it countless benefits for the body, the mind, and, I venture, the soul.

Even those who have already approached these martial arts can find what is presented in Accept the Force of Gravity useful. The detailed explanations of the exercises, and the cards with drawings, allow one to review and possibly correct postures, gestures, breathing, fundamental aspects. To learn well, in fact, the key word is repetition.

Western science has long since discovered contrary to what was believed for decades that it is possible to begin learning something new even at a very advanced age. It is necessary to create new neural pathways, and repetition is the tool through which this "magic" occurs.

The force of gravity the protagonist of the title is the most surprising part, because the way it is explained by Andrea, and the meaning it has in Taichi and Qigong, turns the common view of it upside down, elevating it to a crucial element for the flow of life energy, Chi, in our body Its meaning expands and now includes, along with the idea of heaviness, its opposite, lightness. The reader is invited first to be aware of its constant action on the body, and to welcome this kind of wave instead of undergoing it to perceive it and cooperate with it to achieve our well-being on multiple levels.

Above all, Andrea was able to make a "serious" topic extremely "light". This aspect alone, in my opinion, makes the book worth reading.

I, however, must admit that I read it first and foremost for love. But this is another book.

Happy reading!
Sara

*Sara Della Bruna, Director and Owner of the B&B Cuore Alpino, Coach Consultant in the psychosocial field, and expert in tourism, began her professional career as a communication manager of an important consumer cooperative society and continued her personal journey with the opening of the Xké Cultural Center, where she developed a passion for the world of frontier science and quantum theories.*

*Since 2022, she has been successfully running the B&B Cuore Alpino in Olivone, in the heart of the Swiss Alps, where, in just a few years, she has created a network of important contacts in the world of psycho-physical well-being, hosting dozens from groups of various spiritual disciplines and cultural backgrounds from Switzerland and other parts of the world; At the same time she has managed to make the B&B Cuore Alpino a reference structure for corporate retreats, tourist stays, and sports internships.*

*A great lover of animals, she is lucky enough to be accompanied by Chanel, a beautiful, faithful, and admirable Labrador.*

*Recognized for her great empathy and passion for hospitality, Sara Della Bruna is considered an example to follow.*

## Coach Mike Cunliffe

### The force of gravity in sport

The book you are about to read is a profound work in the understanding of health and peak human performance. Having coached at the highest levels and having had the privilege of working with the most innovative biohackers, body workers and scientists in the world, I've learned that the keys to living with pinnacle health are to have the body as neutral to gravity as possible combined with maximal cellular integrity. Andrea Laffranchini who I consider a friend and brother, has unlocked a secret and complex mystery which few understand and even fewer know how to obtain.

Andrea shares with you his journey and more importantly his knowledge regarding the cornerstone of the body's neutral relationship to gravity and how to apply it to living in this beautiful world.

To Andrea and to all who read this work "Evviva la vita".

**Coach Mike**

*Coach Mike Cunliffe is widely regarded as one of the world's top power and speed coaches. He holds the highest certifications globally as a World Athletics Level 5 High Performance Coach in sprints and a USATF Level 3 High Performance Coach in sprints.*

*With over two decades of experience, he has pioneered the integration of structural optimization aligning the body's natural relationship to gravity and cellular optimization combined with USATF Olympic training protocols at the highest levels of international track and field. His expertise in tailoring training to each athlete's Event Specific Demand (ESD) has propelled his athletes to compete in multiple Olympic Games, as well as World Junior/U20 and World Youth/U18 Championships, representing over a dozen nations.*

## Dr. Jyun Shimizu

### Quantum perspective on the force of Gravity

The quantum perspective on gravity, when integrated with the dynamic view, emphasizes not only the subjective experience of gravitational forces but also how these experiences may be influenced by the underlying quantum nature of the universe. Rather than seeing gravity simply as a physical force acting uniformly on all objects, this perspective suggests that gravity is intertwined with the quantum fabric of spacetime, which can be influenced by consciousness and perception.

From this viewpoint, gravity is not just a constant force; it is a dynamic interaction with our physical bodies, consciousness, and the quantum field. The sensation of weight, for example, may fluctuate not only due to our emotional state, activity level, or environment but also based on the quantum fluctuations of spacetime itself. This means that the way we experience gravity can be influenced by the interconnectedness of all things at a quantum level.

Furthermore, the dynamic perspective considers how gravity shapes our relationship with the world in ways that go beyond mere physical interactions. It affects how we navigate spaces, interact with others, and conceptualize our place in the universe, possibly even influenced by quantum entanglement or the observer effect. In this way, gravity is not just a scientific principle but a lived experience that intertwines with our perceptions, emotions, and interactions, shaped by both classical and quantum influences, ultimately guiding our existence as human beings.

Dr. Jyun

*With over 30 years of experience in integrative medicine and quantum principle applications. Dr. Jyun is a leader in sports performance and healing. He has lectured at universities, local communities, and corporate organizations globally and has authored several best-selling books. He actively researches ancient and modern science with technologies to help upgrade human performance and optimization.*

# Introduction

January 2025, I have instinctively decided to go to China to make a Taichi course. I barely knew what it was. The suggestion came from a wonderful person whom I had met a few months earlier. To make a long story short, this person gave me some resources to help heal my body and suggested decreasing my sports activity in favor of martial arts such as Taichi. It was the first time I had heard about it. I'm the kind of person who likes to have new experiences. I downloaded a few Taichi exercises from youtube, practiced them for a few weeks, and very soon have decided to look for a Taichi school in China. That day I was lucky because I immediately fell in love with one of the first centers I found online. About 60 days later I was on the plane to China.

I then decided to put on paper this amazing one-month experience. I was not, and I am not, an expert in Taichi or Qigong and for that very reason, I have tried to write in a simple and comprehensive way what it is all about.

**Everything I write is what I have heard and learned from the outstanding teacher, Master Ping. I haven't copied anything from books or from the internet. I have only quoted a few sentences from the sheets that Master Ping made available at the FangYuanTaiChi Center.**

Everything you read here is simply my experience in Chaochan, China, in April 2025.

There may be some inaccuracies in what I write, but I don't think it is relevant to the purpose of this book.

**I aim to spark the interest and curiosity of as many people as possible because I'm truly convinced that Qigong and Taichi are practices that awaken self-care and a deeper awareness of our body and our soul.**

You will find a detailed explanation of how to perform Qigong and Taichi exercises. I don't think you'll find much literature that goes into such detail. The reason may be that it's not easy to explain every single movement in words. I tried to write out each movement of some Qigong and Taichi forms because doing so helped me while learning during my intensive one-month course. I therefore suggest that anyone who wants to start practicing Qigong or Taichi should first do the exercises with a trainer and, after repeating each exercise at least 15 to 20 times, read through my detailed explanations. There may be some imperfections, but if so, they are not relevant and do not prevent a critical and constructive reading of one's own progress.

# My travel to China

It was finally time to check in online, on the morning of the day of my departure. It had been a busy week, and I did not have much time to concentrate on the detailed aspects of my trip despite Sara having asked me several times if I had organized everything. I called the airline's customer service to get help to complete the transaction as it did not seem to go smoothly. 'The trip has been booked for March 27th' the consultant repeated to me twice. Impatiently, I confirmed to her and asked again why it was not possible to check in for my flight. Sara, sitting next to me, looked at me and said 'Andrea, today is March 28th'

Everything worked out and a few hours later we were at Bellinzona station. It was forty-five minutes before the train left. As we ordered a coffee, I imagined myself pulling my card out of my pocket, when she placed an envelope, a postcard and a lucky charm on the table.

'I wish you something serious, lightness. Suddenly over 27 years of growing love passed through my head. I decided to place my envelope on the table as well. We looked at each other intensely.

She was feverish, so I urged her not to wait for the train to arrive. I had not thought about the journey and its preparation, but I imagined many times our greeting, me from the train and her from the platform.

I waited about ten minutes and published on Instagram the lyrics accompanied by an excerpt of a Giovanotti song, "To you".

I barely saw Hong Kong, just enough time to go out for a tea. I got up at five in the morning to avoid making Master Ping's driver wait in vain a second time at Chaochan station.

Twenty-four hours later, at five fifty-five in the morning of March 30th, 2025, I entered China. The immigration procedure took an hour and already made me understand how I was entering another world.

Arriving at the train station, after showing my passport three times, completing a series of administrative procedure and above all surviving the customs officer's rather forceful request to put my fingers on the device to register my fingerprints, I joined the queue standing in front of a gate. The sign stated the rule to go to the platform only 15 minutes before the departure of the trains. We silently and diligently made our way to the train cars.

The first class was quiet and tidy. Adjacent to the lavatory there was a rather large faucet with a mirror, shelf and a vase of fresh flowers that contrasted with the grayness of the environment perceived up to that moment.

We spent a good half hour in the tunnel, I imagined crossing the sea surrounding Hong Kong. The landscape suddenly presented itself exactly as my imagination had visualized it. Huge colorless buildings, clustered together and vast land cultivated with rice.

At the first stop my attention was caught by the rows of people standing on the platform in order one behind the other. Four or five rows waiting for the train and ready to get on. I imagined the kids intent on learning at school the rules of good behavior inherited from the communist regime.

At the second stop, a distinguished gentleman sat down next to me, apparently not very nice. I glanced at him discreetly from time to time, but he did not even hint at a smile. Ten minutes later in a totally unexpected manner, he asked me where I was from. 'Is that in Europe?' he asked me sharply. 'Sweden?' he asked me a second time. I showed him on the map of the world downloaded from the internet where Switzerland is. With a smile he said "Geneva?". I gave him a knowing look and he proudly told me about cheese and the Swiss Army knife.

I inserted my passport in the gate and looked for Mr. Ping's driver who had not replied to my message informing him of my arrival. Compared to the day before when he had made the journey in vain, the chauffeur was not there. I sent a message to Mister Ping without success.

I decided to have a coffee and waited for his call hoping it would come before my phone's battery died.

The young lady at the counter looked at me smiling. After typing a few words on her phone, she asked me in robotic English which coffee I wanted. The menu in Mandarin was incomprehensible to me. I typed on her phone 'ristretto coffee'.

I imagine her surprise on my absurd request. She offered me an American coffee. I still couldn't imagine that they didn't accept Hong Kong dollars. I went out to look for an ATM, but I discovered quickly that there were none.

I finally found a girl who spoke English and asked her if there was an exchange office. I imagine because of the disappointment, she took out her bag a hundred renminbi, which I later discover was enough for a coffee but also for lunch. I looked at her with surprise and decisively refused her offer. She insisted. I then decided to gamble the few minutes left of my cell phone battery by looking in internet for the exchange rate with the Hong Kong dollar and handed her the equivalent of what she kindly offered me. I evidently rejected her proposal to give me the difference.

I re-entered the cafeteria proudly displaying the one hundred renminbi note when I was surprised to hear a sentence that certainly didn't taste like coffee. While I was about to leave, I was invited to sit down. A few minutes later, I have got a hot American coffee. At my gesture to pay, I received a nod of refusal.

Two hours have passed since my message to Master Ping and my phone had thirty percent battery left.

I decided to eat something.

I entered for the second time the take-away that I had previously visited in vain in my second attempt to get a coffee with Hong Kong dollars. This time I entered with pride, showing the legendary banknote still intact.

The smiles of the numerous employees who looked at each other for approval let me know that I could pay for my upcoming meal with peace of mind.

I ordered my meal from one of the numerous and incomprehensible drawings accompanied by their equally incomprehensible written description. While I felt the curious looks of the other customers I enjoyed my first meal in China.

Now confident, I visited a third takeaway, ordered a second coffee and made friends with a lady who was also waiting to receive hers. Maybe the word friendship is a little rash, but these brief dialogues introduced me gently and pleasantly to this new reality.

Just before the phone's battery was drained, I got the phone call I was waiting for. The driver was on his way.

After about 20 minutes and about ten kilometers, leaving the dreary, gray main road, we entered a side street surrounded by flowering plants that seemed to welcome me. Suddenly the gray sky appeared to gentle me and of a welcoming color.

After forty-eight hours of traveling and over eight thousand kilometers, I was welcomed into the magical structure which seemed even more beautiful and harmonious than I had imagined.

I experienced a feeling of happiness. After a short round of inspection, I fell asleep.

I found myself running with some local kids who, amused, accompanied me barefoot the first ten meters of my repeats. I found myself answering a boy sitting on a motorbike behind a girl who, after pronouncing his name, asked me with gestures for mine. I was doing my first running training on another planet, with an audience of onlookers who made me realize how we in Western Countries have lost simplicity and spontaneity. It was not a dream, it was reality.

I thought of Sara's wish for something serious, called lightness, that in that moment felt so true to me, but which I didn't yet know would turn out to be even more surprising.

# Qi, our vital energy

## The meridians

To better understand Qigong and Taichi philosophy it is important to understand the meridians which, simply put, are the "transport system" of your life energy throughout the body and organism. Meridians are the circulatory system of energy that works like the circulatory system of blood, but instead of blood they transport the Qi ("chee"), which is our life energy, without which we could not live.

It is not an easy concept to explain and there are several elements that need to be considered, such as the number of meridians, the direction of energy flow, Yin and Yang duality, bridging and more. The meridians are connected to our organs such as the stomach, bladder, gallbladder, large and small intestines, liver, spleen, kidneys, and lungs.

Altogether, there are 26 long meridians, 12 on the right side of our body, 12 on the left side, and 2 additional ones, Du and Rèn. These are the meridians people are most familiar with. Some of these meridians correspond to a specific major organ. All the major meridians pass through a peripheral flap, a hand or a foot. From there, each channel travels either up or down the body.

As part of a larger universe, meridians bridge the gap between our small universe – the body -and the Qi, or energy. Through the use of various practices, including acupuncture, massage, exercises, diet, herbal remedies, Qigong and Taichi, this vital energy system is controlled to promote health.

Compared to traditional Western medicine, the "Chinese medicine" is a holistic model and is related to nature. Dysfunction and disease are not seen as the result of pathology but as imbalances in the Qi and other energetic systems.

## Meridians in Qigong and Taichi

The body is our little universe, just as the environment around us is the big universe. As the universe is always moving, our body has also to move. That's why we say that sitting is the second way of smoking. Sitting doesn't make our internal energy move, and the body creates a lot of negative energy. It is therefore important to let the vital energy, the Qi, flow up into our spine because our energy channel is connected to the spine.

In Qigong and in Taichi there is a lot of stretching of the spine and back exercises to create a smooth flow of energy. Since energy must circulate in the entire body from the head to the feet it is important to stretch the spine and there are different exercises in both Qigong and Taichi. There is for example the first *brocade lifts up the hands to regulate the sinjiao* or the second brocade *drawing the bow to shoot the eagle*, or the second Taichi, *the taichi circle.*

The spine is only one important part of the energy circulation. Every single part of our body contributes to it and these extraordinary disciplines offer exercises to give the body the flow it needs. Let's take for example the Qigong and the Baduanjin, in English the 8 brocades. In all eight of these exercises there are a lot of benefits like improving the blood and energy circulation, strengthening the shoulders and the arms, increase lung capacity, open the chest area, balance the spleen and stomach, enhance digestion, relax the neck, ease eye fatigue, regulate liver energy, calm emotion, alleviate stress, strengthen the kidneys and enhance lower limb flexibility, increase limb strength, relieve stress, promote circulation and clearing energy channels.

All these energy channel circulates through the meridians. One example is the meridian in our back that starts from the perineum and rises to the top of the head and descends to the mouth. In Chinese it is called the *du* meridian. The *pelvic moving warm* up exercises activate all entire energy channel. The same logic applies to the meridian that runs from the mouth down to the pelvic floor, in Chinese the *Rèn* meridian. These two meridians are very important in the Chinese philosophy.

The *du* meridian (back) is the Yang while the *Rèn* meridian (front) is the Yin. Yin, which is typically passive, feminine and associated with the moon, is contrasted with Yang, which is active, masculine and related to the sun. It is curious to know that Yang is in the back because the the animals' backs, as they walk, are in the direction of the sun (see black and sun), while Yin is in the front of the animal because as they walk they are in the direction of the ground (see white and moon). The same applies to other meridians. For example, the meridian that goes from the thumb to the shoulder is the Yang because it is facing the sun.

Let's show how Qigong exercise can help activate a meridian. The *drawing the bow to shoot the eagle* exercise stimulates the lung energy channel because it stretches the upper part of the arm to the thumb (see the thumb position of this exercise) which corresponds to the meridian that goes, on the outside from the shoulder to the thumb, while inside even deeper to the lung.

Qigong practices get the energy flowing again and improve and benefit the respective organs. Each exercise has different specific benefits for different parts of the body or soul. Some parts of the body and soul can receive benefits from different Qigong or Taichi exercises. Lung capacity also benefits from the *look back to release tension and fatigue* exercise.

Another example is the liver which is known to be related to emotions. If you are not in a good mood all this negative energy gets stuck in the liver region. The *separate the hands to regulate the spleen and the stomach Qigong exercise* is also functional to remove the blockage and make the energy channel in that meridian flow again.

People who don't sleep well are advised to unlock the back meridian that runs from the foot to the back, the neck and the top of the head through the *sway the head and wag the tail to release heart fire* exercise.

Moving, stretching, flowing are the way to open the blocked energy channel.

# Reverse Breathing

Breathing plays a very important role in Qigong and Taichi. There may be other theories on how to breathe, but I would like to focus on breathing during the Qigong and Taichi exercises.

However, in the initial phase of learning, it is better not to pay too much attention to how to breathe. Rather, it is recommended to focus on how to perform the exercises. Once you are more familiar with them, you can start thinking about how to breathe. Master Ping focused on reverse breathing.

Reverse breathing means that when you inhale you need to pull your belly in, while when you exhale you must push it out. When you inhale, you must imagine having a ball in your belly that becomes smaller, while when you exhale you must imagine a swelling ball.

It is also important to use the nose and not the mouth, so as not to block the energy connection coming down from the back of the head through the face. An open mouth would block the flow of energy. To make the energy flow downwards even better, it is important to raise the tongue until it touches the palate. Doing this gesture during the exercise allows the brain to memorize it until it becomes a habit.

You will find instructions on how to breathe in the meditation chapter, as well as in the chapters dedicated to the Qigong and Taichi exercises.

# Massage tapping

In China there are different ways to unblock energy channels. Apart from Taichi and Qigong, there are other practices such as massages, aquapuncture, various methods of stretching the body, breathing, cup massage, Gua sha, tapping massage, soft hammer, comb massage, and so on. I will focus on the soft hammer, palm, comb and hand self-massage.

## Soft hammer

The soft hammer is a therapy that can be done by everyone on their own with a special "soft hammer". It is a wonderful tool that is done with the mugwort plant (Artemisia vulgaris). The purpose is to make the energy of the body circulate through different meridians. For example, to increase the lung capacity, you need to work on the meridian that runs from the shoulder to the thumb. It is necessary to start tapping the soft hammer on the shoulder muscle in a repetitive, constant and firm manner and go down through the meridian to the thumb, passing by the pectoral muscle, the armpit, the deltoid, the biceps muscle, the forearm muscles, to the palm. You tap a little bit on the right and on the left. It is important you stay on the front part of the arm because the direction of the tapping must correspond to the direction of Qi (energy) circulation. Once you have tapped all your front part of the arm, you do the same on the other arm and repeat the procedure.

You can then move on to the back of the arm starting from the back of the hand to the trapezius. This meridian is good for digestion and the health of the small and large intestines.

You can then start with another part of the body.

We divide the body into 5 sections. The arms, the legs, the spine, the front part of the torso and the head.

The soft hammer can be used for the arms, the legs, the spine.

As a reminder you must tap from top to bottom all over the body except the back of the arm, the back of the leg and the inner side of the leg where you must tap from bottom to top.

In general, where you have big muscles, you can tap harder and where you have small muscles softer.

The hammer will become softer as you use it.

## Cuppy palm

The front part of the body (chest to belly) can't be tapped with the soft hammer because there is not enough flesh. This is the reason why we can use the palm of the hand, which must be bent forward (cup-shaped palm). You can tap regularly and firmly from the top to bottom on the left, on the center and on the right side of the front of the body. This is also beneficial for highly emotional people, because the meridians of the emotions are located there. While tapping, you can let out the 'aaaah' sound from your mouth to let out negative emotions.

## Comb massage

Moodiness, fatigue, excessive stress, hair loss, insomnia, headaches could be related to the lack of energy circulation also in the head where several meridians are also located.

One way to unblock the energy channel is to use a special wooden comb.

There are many benefits such as increasing blood circulation, reducing stress and tension, increasing sleep quality, preventing hair loss, enhancing mental clarity, relieving headaches and alleviating migraine.

In particular, head massage stimulates Qi flow and improves blood circulation by reducing blockages and promoting overall vitality. By targeting pressure points and easing muscle tension, head massage can provide relief from headaches and migraines and improve physical comfort. It stimulates blood flow to the scalp, which can nourish hair follicles and prevent hair loss. It helps release tension, promoting relaxation and better sleep. Stimulating acupressure points on the scalp can improve mental clarity and focus.

One should start at the centre line of the head from the top front to the back, exerting good pressure on the comb in an as if combing, but with more pressure act to combing but stronger. You must do it 36 times.

You do the same on the sides as well as on the lower lines of the head. It is beneficial for sleeping and reducing stress as well as for digestion and reducing toxins of the body.

Afterwards, the sequence is repeated but moving the comb quickly to the right and left following the centre line, the upper side and the lower side of the head.

If your head feels a little sore, this means that some points are blocked, and the massage aims precisely at unblocking them.

With another part of this comb, you can also massage the ear and eyes.

## Hand massage

To complete the body massage, one can finally move on to the face and neck. One method consists of rubbing your hands together, massaging them with good energy and then massaging your face in various places and directions. One can also massage the belly with firm, multi-directional movements. It aids digestion.

I would like to reiterate how this type of massage, in addition to unblocking energy, makes the muscle fascia more flexible, the muscle stronger, and offers a number of additional health benefits.

Master Ping suggests doing self-massage once per day.

# Meditation

## What it is about

In order to understand what meditation is about, it is important to understand a few concepts.

In the body we have three points that are not organs, muscles, bones or anything else. They are energy. The lower Dantian, the center of energy, the middle Dantian, the center of breathing and the upper Dantian, the center of concentration. In the physiology of traditional Chinese Medicine, the place in the body where Qi is stored, accumulated, and from where it then radiates into the different meridians of the body.

In Qigong, Taichi and meditation practices, there are some exercises where you need to keep Qi exactly in front of the lower and middle Dantian.

If you hold Qi in the lower Dantian you are holding the internal life energy, while if you are holding Qi in the middle Dantian you are holding the energy of the environment.

Another important concept is the *Bai Hui* and *Hui Yin* points in the body. The *Bai Hui* is located on the top of the head while the *Hui Yin* is located on the bottom of the pelvis. When stretching the upper back, it helps to visualise your *Bai Hui,* and when stretching the lower back it helps to visualise your *Hui Yin.*

The two very important meridians of the body, the *Du* meridian and the *Ren* meridian help the energy to rise to the *Bai Hui* when you inhale and to descend to the *Hui Yin* when you exhale.

This concept is fundamental to performing Qigong, Taichi and meditation exercises correctly. One must think of the body as a puppet suspended and attached to the head and other parts of the body, depending on the movements one is doing.

"A Puppet that is firmly rooted to the ground through the front/center of the feet that must carry and accept the force of gravity and return it to the body upwards" This concept inspired me to coin a motto that I make my own and which becomes the basis of our well-being and the title of this book: **accept the force of gravity**. A concept that, if understood and put into practice, can also help in sport but especially in everyday life.

This type of meditation is not aimed at achieving a hypnotic state but is functional in helping the consciousness to move life energy, which in turn helps move the body. It is a matter of being able to focus attention on the inside of the body and on sharing it with the force of gravity. Meditation is about balancing the bone structure to make it stronger as well as tendons and ligaments more elastic, it is about relaxing the body and the muscles. It is about making the body more sensitive, to allow it to think about our small universe. Once you can do that, you will automatically be connected to the big universe because everything is connected. It takes a little time. Don't worry, don't rush it.

Meditation can have many benefits, but only if you do it correctly and consistently:

- Opens energy channels
- Relaxes
- Primarily strengthens the bone structure
- Gives a correct posture

Doing it daily for about 20 minutes will help to get to know the body and its strengths better. It will help to connect to the small universe, to better feel the circulation of life energy, to understand if and where there may be blockages that do not allow Qi to circulate properly. Meditation is the basis for performing Qigong and Taichi exercises in the best possible way.

## How to do it

1. Find your centre line: you must first focus on your body position. Your shoulders should be aligned with your feet.

2. Stretch the upper spine: you need to focus on the *Dai Hui* – the top of your head – and try to stretch your spine upwards while keeping your chin facing forward and pull the *Dai Hui* upwards

3. Relax your muscles: try to relax all the muscles in your body, starting from your shoulder to the rest of your body

4. Stretch your lower spine: bend your knees, move your pelvis slightly forward, and imagine you are pulling your *Hui Yin* downwards.

5. Stretch the entire spine, upwards the *Dai Hui* and downwards the *Hui Yin.*

6. Put your full body weight on your feet: imagine you're hanging from a nail with your full body weight on your feet. 70% of the weight should be on the middle/front of the feet (the remaining 30% on the rest of the feet)

7. Raise your arms: bring your arm up to Qi at chest height – the middle Dantian. The elbow should be bent at 90 degrees, detach the upper arm from the torso. Now the arms are connected to the upper spine as well as the legs are connected to the lower spine.

8. Stay in this position for at least ten minutes listening to your body, spine and all the steps I have just explained above

9. Bring your lower arm down towards the lower Dantian and hold Qi

10. Bring your arms down near your sides with your palms facing down

11. Start breathing in, inhaling as you raise your hands up to chest level, lifting your legs slightly. As you inhale, imagine that your head, middle palm, anus, and tops of your feet are also inhaling. Exhale by bringing your hands

and legs down, imagining that you are exhaling with the other part of the body just described. Repeat as many times as you feel it

12. Bring your arms up to chest height and hold your Qi. Start breathing in, inhaling as you open your arms outward while lifting your legs slightly. As you inhale, imagine that your head, middle palm, anus, and the tops of your feet are also inhaling. Exhale by bringing the hands back to hold the Qi and the legs down, imagining that you are exhaling with the other part of the body just described. Repeat as many times as you feel like.

13. Bring your arms back close to your sides with your palm facing downwards. Open your hand and close it as if your hand were breathing. Start breathing and bring your hands and the air over your head. Return downwards while exhaling. Repeat as many times as you feel.

14. Make three circles with your hands and at the fourth circle hold Qi at chest level

15. Bring your hands close to your hips, close your left leg, put your left arm on your stomach and your right hand on your left hand (the opposite if you are a woman) and bend your torso forward.

Concentrate on everything your body needs to do to be able to relax. During meditation, it would be helpful to have a person to guide you and tell you what you need to do, step by step.

We recommend one session a day of 30 minutes:

- 5' find the right position – point 1 to 6 above
- 15' hold Qi – points 7 and 8 above
- 10' breathing – point 9 to 14 above

Keep your fingers slightly open (maximum a couple of cm between the fingers) but relaxed, palm slightly arched. When you breathe try to feel your breathing pass through your fingertips (tingling) and the centre of your hand.

# Warm-up exercises

**Before each Qigong or Taichi session, it is important to warm up the body for about 10 minutes. Here is a possible warm-up session.**

## Neck

1. Stand straight with your body and bend your knees slightly to find the right balance. Bring your neck up and forward, descend with your chin towards the lower part of your neck, touch your neck and start the circular movement again. Repeat 16 more times.

2. Stand straight with your body and bend your knees slightly to find the right balance.

3. Do the same movements as above, but in the opposite direction. Repeat 16 more times.

## Shoulders

1. Stand straight with your body bending slightly your knees to find the right balance.

2. Spin your arms like a windmill first in one direction for 16 times and then in the other direction for 16 times.

3. Stand straight with your body bending slightly your knees to find the right balance.

4. Swing your right arm slightly laterally and upward (slightly raising your right foot) and your left arm slightly laterally and backwards then swing your left arm slightly laterally and upwards (slightly raising your left foot) and your right arm slightly laterally and backwards for about 16 times.

Do the same exercise but continue the movement of both hands above your head until you touch both your hands (it is good if you hear the sound).

## Lower back

1. Stand straight with your body bending slightly your knees to find the right balance.

2. Rotate your pelvis to the left in a circular motion 16 times. Change direction.

3. Stand straight with your body bending slightly your knees to find the right balance.

4. Rotate your tailbone to the left in a circular motion 16 times.

Change direction.

5. Stand straight with your body bending slightly your knees to find the right balance.

6. Rotate your pelvis on the left and on the right letting arms follow in the same direction and letting the hands touch the buttocks for 16 times.

7. Rotate your pelvis to the left and right letting arms follow in the same direction and letting the hands touch the back at navel level, 16 times.

8. Rotate your pelvis to the left and right letting arms follow in the same direction and letting the hands touch the back at shoulder level 16 times

## Legs

1. Step forward with the left foot, bring the right knee forward and upwards and roll it to the right, rest it back in the starting position, bring your left foot back to the starting position 16 times. Repeat this sequence 16 times.

2. Step forward with your right foot, bring the left knee forward and up and swing it to the left, rest it in the starting position, bring the right foot back to the starting position 16 times.

3. Do the same exercise but move your right knee in the opposite direction, from side to front and back to the starting position 16 times.

4. Do the same exercise but move your left knee in the opposite direction, from side to front and back to the starting position 16 times.

5. Put your right foot in front of your left foot and lift your left leg sideways as high as you can without forcing. Once back at the starting position do the same on the other side, lifting your right leg sideways. Repeat this sequence 16 times.

6. Put your left foot forward and move your right leg as if you were kicking a ball. Once back put your right foot forward and move your left leg as if you were kicking a ball. Repeat this sequence 16 times.

## Two hands hold the feet to strengthen the kidneys and waist

Finish the warmup session with the brocade no.6 for 6 times – see instructions below.

# Qigong

Baduanjin is a traditional Qigong practice that consists of eight individual movements. Known for its simplicity, natural flow and ease of learning, each movement incorporates stretching chest expansion and rotation to help circulate energy and blood throughout the body, improve flexibility and balance, strengthen muscles and joints, and enhance internal organ function and circulation. Due to its practicality, Baduanjin has become a popular choice for office workers seeking to relieve stress and improve sub-health conditions.

Baduanjin is also known as "the 8 brocades".

## Benefits of Qigong

As a traditional exercise method, it has significant health benefits, making it especially suitable for office workers who spend long hours at their desks, each specific benefit includes:

1. Relieves neck and shoulder stiffness: long hours at the computer can lead to neck and shoulder tension. The *drawing the bow to shoot the eagle* movement helps relax this area through gentle stretching.

2. Reduces lower back pressure: prolonged sitting can cause lower back discomfort. *Two hands hold the feet to strengthen the kidneys, and the waist,* effectively exercises the lower back muscle, easing strain on the back.

3. Improves blood circulation: deep breathing combined with the movements accelerates blood flow, helping to relieve cold hands and feet.

4. Improves concentration and reduces stress: these rhythmic low movements and breathing patterns can improve mood, reduce anxiety and increase concentration.

5. Promote digestion: The *separate hands to regulate the spleen and stomach* movement improve digestive function, benefiting those who suffer from poor digestion due to prolonged sitting.

## Qigong exercises

Preamble: holding Qi means placing your hands in front of your body in the indicated position as if you were holding and hugging a large ball touching your arms and chest.

### Two hands lift up to regulate SanJiao – n.1

1. Put the legs together
2. Bend your knees
3. Open the left leg with legs at shoulder level
4. Rotate your arms up and down in a circular motion three times moving your head back slightly as you raise your arms
5. The fourth time bring your hands down back at pelvis level and make a small circle to hold them at chest height – hold the Qi
6. Lower your hands to the pelvis and hold the Qi
7. Bring the hands together with the palm up, crossing the fingers
8. Bring the hands up to chest height
9. "Turn the hands 360 degrees" and continue the movement over the head as high as you can, while you throw your head backwards.
10. Straighten your head
11. Lower your arms just above your head

12. Release your hands and bring them back to the height of your pelvis with a circle
13. Hold Qi at pelvis level
14. Repeat the sequence from n. 8 for 6 times
15. Hold Qi at pelvis level

### Drawing the bow to shoot the eagle – n. 2

1. Shift your weight onto your right leg and move your left leg 20cm to 30cm to the left
2. Bend your knees and raise your hands next to the body to create a cross – the left hand must be on the outside
3. Turn your pelvis and your head to the left, extending the left hand to the left, moving the right hand with the elbow bent to the right keeping it resting on the chest, until you reach the position of a man about to shoot an arrow with a drawn bow. Make a fist with your left hand while holding your thumb and index finger up while clenching your right hand like a claw
4. Raise your right forearm until your arm is straight and parallel to your left arm, while turning your head back in the center
5. Turn your left foot forward, bring back to the center your left leg to the starting position while bringing your hands back
6. Hold the Qi at chest level
7. Repeat the entire exercise on the other side
8. Repeat the two sequences 3 times
9. Move back your feet at starting position, hold the Qi at pelvis level

### Separate the hands to regulate the spleen and stomach – n.3

1. Move your right hand to the right keeping the palm down until it is located next to the hip, while moving your left palm upwards and when it is at chest height rotate it 360 degrees and extend it as far as possible without forcing. The two hands must be slightly forward

2. Bring back your left hand next to the left hip making the same movement, ending up with the palm down

3. Just before the left hand is next to the hip, start the same sequence with the right hand

4. Repeat the sequence 3 times

5. Finish with arms facing downwards

### Look back to release tension and fatigue – n. 4

1. Move both hands a little bit forward and then back making a circle and keeping them at pelvis level while turning them until your palm faces towards, move back both your shoulders, move your chest forward as you turn your head to the left until you look backward

2. Bring your head, chest, shoulder and hand back to the starting level

3. Repeat the exercise to the right

4. Repeat the sequence 3 times

5. Hold Qi at pelvis level

### Sway the head and wag the tail to release heart fire – n. 5

1. Shift your weight to your right leg and move your left leg 20cm to 30cm to the left

2. Move both hands upwards vertically, keeping them close to each other, until they extend above your head and bring them back down laterally forming a circle until they rest on your legs
3. Bend your left knee forward while extending your right leg and turn your pelvis on the left
4. Create an arc in your back as you approach your left foot and look at your left foot
5. Extend your left leg by bending your right knee, straighten your back by moving it to the right, moving your neck to the right, continuing looking at your left foot until your neck is aligned with your left leg and your trunk
6. Move your perineum to the left, then forward, then to the right and as you move it back move at the same time your neck from the right to the back
7. Move your neck forward while bending your knees
8. Extend your knees
9. Repeat the same exercise on the other side
10. Repeat the sequence 3 times
11. Bring back your left leg to the right
12. Hold Qi at pelvis level

### Two hands hold the feet to strengthen the kidneys and waist – n.6

1. Rotate your arms outward and upward like a circle and bring them back down vertically next to the hip with your palm facing downwards
2. Raise your hands above the head vertically

3. When they are above your head, lower them by holding the palm downwards at chest height and bring back the head at initial position

4. Turn both palms upwards, slide your hands behind your back holding them against your body

5. Place the palm of your hand against your body, straighten your legs and slide your hands down your back, your back and legs to the ankles and down to touch your foot while keeping your back slightly bent at the top

6. Slightly bend your head forward, arch your back up, extend your hands and bring your back up again while keeping both your back and hand outstretched

7. Repeat the exercise from n.2 for 6 more times

8. Bring your hands back at pelvis level and hold Qi

**Clench fists with eyes glared fiercely to build strength and Qi – n.7**

1. Open your left leg of about 20cm to 30cm and make a fist in both hands with the thumb inside the fist, while holding your fingers towards the body

2. Move your left arm forward and stretch-in it in front of your body

3. Rotate the fist to the right as far as you can

4. Open your hand and rotate it by stretching it towards your body, to the left until it has your palm facing upward

5. Close your hand again forming a fist and bring your arm back to your side with your finger pointing towards the body

6. Repeat the exercise with the right arm

7. Repeat the sequence 3 times

8. Bring your hands next to the hips holding the palms of the hands facing the ground

### Lifting the heel 7 times keeps 100 illness away – n.8

1. Raise your heels as high as you can without forcing
2. Stay a few seconds
3. Stretch your back upward and relax your lower body imagining yourself suspended in the air
4. Lower your heels halfway keeping them off the ground
5. Stay a few seconds
6. Rest your feet on the ground by slightly forcing the movement, paying attention to the noise your feet make when they touch the ground
7. Repeat the sequence 6 more times (the eighth brocade is the only one you repeat 7 times vs. 6 the first 6 brocades)
8. Bring your left hand on your belly in the Qi area by placing your right hand on top of your left hand (for females, bring your right hand to your belly in the Qi area, placing your left hand on top of your right)
9. Close your legs, bring your hands to your belly as above and bow down

## Qigong benefits for each exercise

### Two hands lift up to regulate SanJiao – n.1

- Key points: stand with feet together, slowly lift both hands from the abdomen to above the head, palms facing upwards, pause briefly, then put down. Repeat six times. .
- Breathing: Inhale when you raise your hands, exhale when you bring your arms back down, or breath naturally.

**Benefits:**

- Extension up to the spinal column.
- Relaxation of the triple burner area (see note at the end of this chapter).
- Improvement of blood and energy circulation
- In Chinese medicine, the triple burner refers to the chest middle abdomen, and lower abdomen.

- Note: keep the spine upright, relax the shoulders and avoid excessive bending.

### Drawing the bow to shoot the eagle – n.2

- **Key points:** one hand assumes a bow-drawing posture while the other mimics drawing a bowstring. Alternate sides. Repeat six times.
- **Breathing:** Inhale while drawing the bow, exhale when releasing.

**Benefits:**

- It strengthens shoulders and arms.
- It increases lung capacity.
- It opens the chest area.

- **Note:** keep steady, avoid swaying, fully extend your arms and follow hand movements with your gaze.

### Separate the hands to regulate the spleen and stomach – n.3

- **Key points:** Lift one hand upward while the other remains down, alternating sides. Repeat six times.
- **Breathing:** Inhale when lifting, exhale when lowering.

**Benefits:**

- It balances the spleen and stomach.
- It enhances digestion.

- **Note:** keep the body stable and shoulders relaxed while lifting.

### Look back to release tension and fatigue – n.4

- **Key points:** open both arms and rotate palms upward, slowly turning the head side to side. Repeat six times.
- **Breathing:** inhale while turning the head, exhale when returning to center.

**Benefits:**

- It relaxes the neck.
- It eases eye fatigue.
- It regulates liver energy.

- **Note:** avoid excessive neck strain; keep the spine straight.

### Sway the head and wag the tail to release heart fire -n.5

- **Key points:** squat down slightly, bending the body and swaying it gently from side to side. Repeat six times.
- **Breathing:** Inhale when lifting to the left, exhale when bending down, inhale when swaying head and tail, and exhale when returning to center.

Benefits:

- It reduces internal heat.
- It calms emotions.

- It alleviates stress.

- **Note:** perform gently and relax the waist.

### Two hands hold the feet to strengthen the kidneys and waist – n.6

- **Key points:** bend forward, reaching hands downward towards the feet. Repeat six times.

- **Breathing:** inhale as arms rise, exhale as they press down, inhale as the hands move from chest to bottom, exhale when hands reach the feet, pause the breath when arms and back flat, inhale when lifting arms, and exhale when pressing down.

**Benefits:**

- It strengthens the kidneys.
- It enhances lower limb flexibility.

- **Note:** avoid forcing yourself too low. Keep relaxed.

### Clench fists with eyes glared fiercely to build strength and Qi – n.7

- **Key points:** clench fists, punch forwards with a fierce look. Repeat six times.

- **Breathing:** inhale while clenching, exhale while punching, inhale when retracting.

**Benefits:**

- It increases limb strength.
- It relieves stress.

- **Note:** maintain even breathing and slight body rotation while punching.

**Lifting the heel 7 times keeps 100 illness away – n.8**

- **Key points:** rise onto tiptoes, then drop heels gently. Repeat seven times.
- **Breathing:** inhale when lifting, exhale when lowering.

**Benefits:**

  - It promotes circulation.
  - It clears energy channels.

- **Note:** rise and fall slightly, keep shoulders relaxed.

## More to know

In general, emphasize natural, relaxed movements, avoid excessive force and maintain a smooth pace. Concentrate, stay calm, and avoid distractions during practice. Increase repetitions gradually to avoid overexertion. Match breathing with movement. Inhale when stretching, exhale when releasing. Adjust intensity and duration based on physical condition. Morning or evening is ideal for practice. Avoid practicing after meals, when overly fatigued, or just before sleeping.

Badunjin is a Qigong health practice suitable for all ages. With daily practice, it helps improve circulation, strengthen the body, relax the mind and promote overall wellness.

*Note from internet: Triple Burner*

*In Chinese, the Triple Burner is known as San Jiao, which is often translated as* "three burning spaces"*. It is also known as the Triple Warmer, Triple Energizer, or the Triple Heater. The Triple Burner is not actually a physical organ (which confuses Westerners). Even academics and/or experts have argued about Triple Burner's true nature. This "non-organ" is believed to consist of several vital body functions. One of its major functions is to regulate the movement of water within the body.*

*Functions of the Triple Burner: You may have heard the Triple Burner referred to as the thermostat of the body, meaning it controls the central heating system. Simply put: the Triple Burner affects the distribution of both body fluids and Qi. Therefore, any dysfunction or blockage in one or more Burners means neither will flow smoothly.*

## Summary Qigong Table - in red the part of the body that benefits most

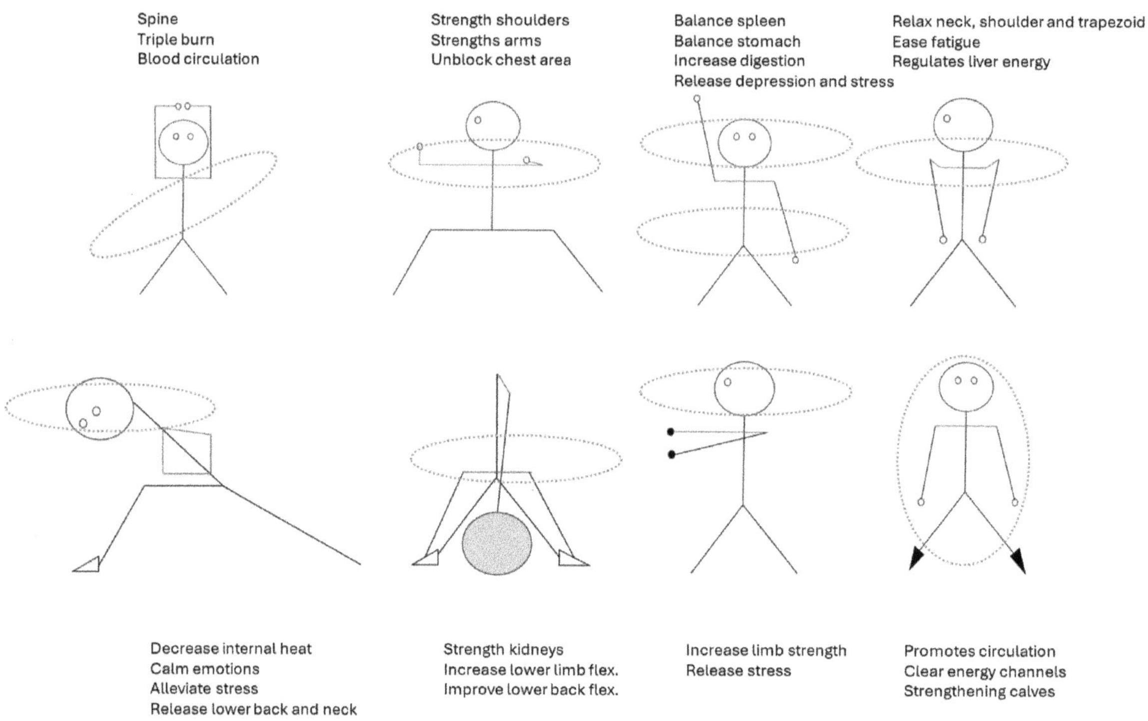

# Taichi

Taichi is a traditional Chinese martial art deeply influenced by philosophy, incorporating elements of martial arts, health practices, Qigong, and philosophy. It aims to regulate the flow of energy, enhance physical fitness, and improve the quality of life through slow, continuous, and graceful movements. Taichi emphasizes the principle of using stillness to control movement and is an art that unites body and mind.

In Daoist philosophy, Taichi refers to the original state of the universe embodying the natural laws of Yin and Yang balance and interdependence of all things. Taichi is not only a philosophical concept but also represents the characteristics of Taichi movements and softness and firmness.

Taichi practice stresses the integration of mind and body. Unique movements and breathing techniques enhance internal strength. Focus is placed on relaxation, roundness, and expansion, achieving coordination of the body, regulation of internal energy, and improvement of immunity through forms, push hands, and other routines.

## Characteristics of Taichi movements

- Gentle and slow movements: Taichi is not about forceful or rapid movements instead, it is about slow and rhythmic motions. It enhances strength and stability through delicate and soft movements rather than relying on quick muscular force.

- Continuous flow: movements are meant to flow continuously like water, emphasizing integration of mind and body, and aiming for natural, fluid motion.

- Breathing and intention: Taichi emphasizes deep abdominal breathing and intention coordination to promote the flow of Qi and blood. Deep breathing enhances oxygen intake, relaxes the body and mind, and regulates energy.

- Yin and Yang transformation: Taichi movements reflect the Daoist concept of Yin and yang, balancing hard and soft, the emptiness and fullness, high and low, fast and slow.

## Benefits of Taichi

- Improving cardiovascular health: Taichi helps increase heart endurance and promotes blood circulation, lowering blood pressure and reducing the risk of heart disease and stroke.

- Enhancing muscle strength and flexibility: Taichi improves muscle strength, especially in the core, while enhancing flexibility and joint mobility.

- Promoting balance and coordination: Taichi improves balance, stability and coordination, reducing the risk of falls, particularly for older adults.

- Regulating breathing and reducing stress: the deep, slow abdominal breathing in Taichi helps regulate Qi and blood flow, relax the body and mind, and alleviate stress.

- Boosting immunity: Taichi enhances immune function by promoting Qi and blood circulation and improving overall metabolism.

- Increasing bone density: weight-bearing movements in Taichi, especially for the lower body, help improve bone health and prevent osteoporosis.

- Promoting Qi circulation and internal organ function: Taichi improves organ function and enhances overall health by stimulating Qi flow through the meridians.

- Relieving pain and preventing chronic disease: Taichi can alleviate pain caused by conditions like arthritis and back pain, and it prevents chronic disease by improving joint function.
- Enhancing mental health and sleep quality: Taichi meditative aspects reduce anxiety and depression, improve sleep quality, and help alleviate insomnia, particularly stress related insomnia.
- Delaying aging and enhancing vitality: Taichi helps maintain vitality by improving circulation and organ function, which delays aging and enhances physical vitality.

## Taichi exercises

### Beginning posture – n.1

1. Put your legs together
2. Bend your knees
3. Open the left leg
4. Raise arms parallel to each other to shoulder height
5. Gently return them to the starting position
6. Repeat the exercise 4 times

### Taichi circle – n.2

1. Bend your elbows while bringing your hands upward keeping your arms adjacent to your torso
2. At chest height cross your arms holding the right one outward
3. Continue the movement with the right arm, while moving back in the opposite direction the left one until completing a full circle while keeping the arms outstretched but light

4. Continue the dynamic movement without stopping for 3 more times while keeping the left arm outside the right arm

5. On the fourth lap stop when the arms are at chest level and start again from step 3 but change direction and keep the left arm outside the right one (after the first lap) for 3 more times

6. Stop when your hands are crossed, move them a little bit forward, breaking the cross and bring them down next to the hips with palms facing down

**Golden rooster – stand on one foot – n.3**

1. Shift your weight onto your left leg and move your right leg next to the left one, placing the tip of the foot on the ground in the 2 o'clock direction, while keeping the knee bent. At the same time move your right hand to the left with the palm upward until it is over your right foot

2. Start moving your right hand upward keeping the palm up and when it is at chest height roll the hand with the palm forward and again upward and extend it as far as possible without forcing, just before your right hand is on top, move up your right leg

3. Bring back your right leg to the ground and your right hand with a vertical movement parallel to your body keeping the palm down

4. Repeat the exercise from n.1 but shift your weight onto your right leg and move your left leg next to the right placing the tip of the foot on the ground in the 10 o'clock direction, and so on

5. Repeat the sequence 4 times

6. Bring your arms next to your hips with your palm down

**Turning the body waving arms – n.4**

1. Turn your torso to the left, bringing your right hand in front of your chest

2. Extend your right arm forward and your left arm back until both arms are stretched and simultaneously turn your head to the left until you are looking backward
3. Bend the elbow of the left arm forward and bring your left hand forward passing next to shoulder height and start turning the head forward
4. Continue the movement of the left arm forward until you are in the same position as the right hand, at the same time bring the right arm back in a movement like stroking a dog until it is stretched behind your body, and at the same time turn your head to the right
5. Repeat the same sequence 3 more times
6. At the eighth sequence while you bring back your right hand towards the left one, when it is stretched forward, bring both hands down next to the pelvis

**Grabs birds' tail on both side – n.5**

1. Turn to the right your right foot at 2 o'clock
2. Move the left leg to the right next to the right leg and rest it with the toe on the ground (empty step) facing 12 o'clock. Simultaneously move your right hand up to the right and your left hand first slightly to the left and then laterally to the right until when they are facing each other aligned with the central part of your body
3. Move your left foot forward and slightly left 20cm or 30cm and bend the knee, keep your bust forward, bring your left hand forward and up to the neck height with the palm facing your body, and your right hand down with the palm facing down
4. Bring the right hand up and to the left next to the left hand

5. Turn both palms in the opposite direction and step down gently to the right by rolling your pelvis in the same direction until you find yourself turned to the right with both hands at the right leg height, while straightening your left knee and bending your right one

6. Place your right hand on the wrist of your left hand and return forward by pushing your left arm with your right hand until you extend it in front of you at chest height, straighten your right knee and bend your left one

7. Finish the movement by bringing the wrist of your right hand slightly over the wrist of your left hand by crossing your hands

8. Open your hands slightly and bring them down close to your thighs by stretching your left leg and bending your right one, move your hands up parallel to your body and push them forward by keeping them at chest height while accompanying your trunk slightly forward stretching your right leg and bending your left knee

9. Bring your left leg back, and your arms horizontally at shoulder level

10. Repeat the same exercise on the other side.

11. Repeat the sequence 4 times

12. Bring your arms next to the hips with palms down

**Kick with Both feet – n.6**

1. Shift your weight onto your left leg and move your right leg next to the left one placing the tip of the foot on the ground in the 2 o'clock direction, while keeping the knee bent

2. Move your arms adjacent to your chest forming a cross with your right hand outward and bring them up over your head until you extend them skyward

3. Move your right leg in a firm upward motion until your right foot touches your right hand that in the meantime you have moved down to the right

4. Hold your arms up and return your leg to the starting position

5. Shift your weight onto your right leg and move your left leg next to the right one placing the tip of the foot on the ground at 10 o'clock direction, while keeping the knee bent

6. Move down both hands to the initial position and move your arms adjacent to your chest forming a cross with your left hand outward and bring them up over your head until you extend them skyward

7. Move your left leg in a firm upward motion until your left foot touches your left hand that in the meantime you have moved down to the left

8. Move down both hands to the initial position

9. Repeat the sequence 3 more times

10. Bring your arms next to the hips with your palm down

### Hold the fist and strike – n.7

1. Shift your weight onto your left leg, bring the right foot next to the left one at 2 o'clock while bringing both your arms next to the flanks making the fists

2. Move your pelvis on the right, take a step forward and to the right with your right foot rested 20cm forward, with the right knee bent forward and the left knee stretched. At the same time move your trunk forward, bend and raise your fists upwards until they are extended and are aligned with your back

3. Bring your arms back bending both elbows until when fists are next to your pelvis

4. Spread your arms outward, roll your shoulders forward bringing your arms upward until they are in line with your back, with the fists' finger pointing externally.

5. Open your fists, stretch your hands backward and rotate them outwards until your palms are facing upward

6. Bring back your arms at pelvis level

7. Turn your pelvis at the initial position

8. Restart from n.1 on the other direction

9. Repeat sequence 4 times

10. Bring your arms next to your hips with your palm down

### Cloudy hands – n.8

1. Lift your left leg and bring it 20 to 30 cm to the left, while lifting your right hand at shoulder level with your palm up and slightly on the right

2. Stretch your left leg and bend your right knee, turn your torso to the right, bring together both hands until the left one is in the central line of your body

3. Move your left hand up and your right hand down

4. Turn both palms to the left, stretch your right leg and bend your left knee, move your bust to the left until the right hand is in the central line of your body

5. Bring up your right hand and down your left

6. Stretch your left leg and bend your right knee, move back your torso to the right turning both palms to the right until when your left hand is in the central line of your body

7. Repeat the sequence 4 times

8. At the 8th movement, stop the sequence when your right arm is in the central line of your body and bring it back to the right at shoulder level and your left hand stays where it is

## Taichi punch – n.9

1. Bring your hands down at pelvic level making fists with both hands with thumb outside fingers and the fingers turned inward

2. Make a firm fist by bringing your right arm forward and rotating your fist so that your fingers point downward, while making a small rotation of your right hip to bring it forward with your arm

3. Return the arm and the fists to the starting position

4. Make a firm fist by bringing your left arm forward and rotating your fist, finding your fingers pointing downward, while making a small rotation of your left hip to bring it forward with your arm

5. Return the arm and the fists to the starting position

6. Repeat the sequence 4 times

7. Bring your arms next to the hips with your palm down

## Closing form – n.10

1. Cross your arms and bring them with the palm facing the bust up in front of your chest keeping your right hand outside

2. Turn your palms outward and then forward and stretch your arms out until they are parallel with each other

3. Bring your arms down next to the hips with a vertical movement

4. Repeat the sequence 4 times

5. Close your left foot

6. Bring up both hands in front of your chest, make a fist with the right hand and open your left hand, beat the fists of the left hand against the palm of the right hand. Bring back both hands next to the hip and lean forward

## More to know

Taichi is not only a martial art form but the practice that promotes physical and mental well-being. Through its gentle movements and deep breathing, it enhances overall health, strengthens the immune system, reduces stress, and improves mental health. Whether for young people or for the elderly, Taichi is an excellent exercise to improve quality of life, prevent disease, and maintain physical health.

## Summary Taichi Table – in red the part of the body that benefits most

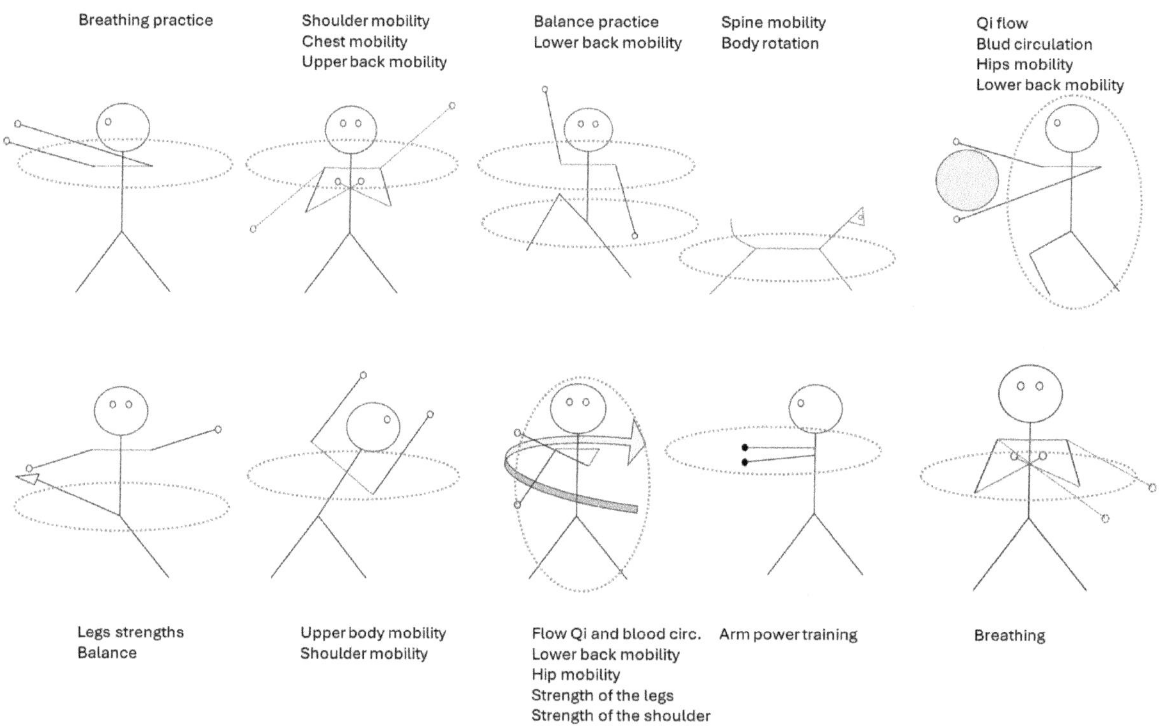

# Similarities and differences between Qigong and Taichi

**Purpose:**

Qigong: health cultivation, body regulation, internal energy training.

Taichi: health, martial arts, self-defense.

**Movements**

Qigong: simple.

Taichi: More complex.

**Breathing**

Qigong: deep, slow abdominal breathing focusing on cultivating internal energy.

Taichi: coordinated with movements, sometimes natural without deliberate control.

**Practice**

Qigong: can be practiced alone or combined with martial arts.

Taichi: primarily through forms and push hands practice.

**Intensity**

Qigong: low intensity, suitable for all age groups.

Taichi: varies from low to high intensity, some martial applications intense.

### Philosophy

Qigong: Daoist health principles, meridian theories.

Taichi: combines Daoist, Confucian and military strategy thoughts, emphasis Yin-Yang transformation.

### Combat

Qigong: non-combat, mainly for self-cultivation.

Taïchi: martial application with combat techniques.

# Combat

To better understand the Taichi movements it is worth spending a few words on the combat technique. It looks like Taichi style has been invented by General Chen in early 1800 who had the idea to merge martial art with Qigong to make soldiers more resistant, strong, healthy and performing for a long time.

The principle of the Taichi combat is to receive the force and to give the force and not struggle against the force. It is the same principle as the force of gravity that must be accepted and let it flow downward into the body to the feet and must be used when it comes up again into the legs, spine and head.

If you are pushed or attacked by a person, you should not resist but make lateral movements or arch your back or abdomen so that you do not counteract the force but accommodate and reuse it to counterattack.

All the Taichi exercise movement apply this principle of receiving the force and giving the force. Concept that is functional for the well-being of the individual and allows better circulation of energy.

To better understand this principle, it would be helpful to simulate during a Taichi course these defense-attack movements.

# Dynamic stretching

Another important tool to better perform Qigong and Taichi exercises is to correctly stretch the body. I would like to share two powerful exercises that enable your body to perform better and to do all the Qigong and Taichi exercises properly.

## Stretch the lower back n.1

**Preparation**

1. Open your legs parallel to your shoulders.
2. Raise your hands to shoulder height.
3. Start the exercise
4. Bend your knees.
5. Rotate your tailbone forward.
6. Bring your hands down close to your pelvis.
7. Stretch your legs.
8. Return the tailbone to the starting position.
9. Raise your hands to shoulder height.

Continue the sequence 30 more times.

This sequence is effective for stretching the back and arms. Specifically:

1. Bend your knees: you relax your body and create the conditions for being able to rotate your pelvis, an operation that would otherwise be impossible.

2. Rotate your tailbone forward: stretch your back.

3. Lower your hands near your pelvis: relax your body.

4. Stretch your legs: stretch your arms and back.

5. Bring the tailbone back to the starting position: relax the body.

6. Raise your hands to shoulder height: the conditions are created for the following movements.

The crucial movement is the rotation of the pelvis. If you can't do it correctly, just practice that movement. Move your arms to your sides and rotate your pelvis back and forth, back and forth 30 times.

## Stretch the lower back n.2

**Preparation**

1. Bring your right leg forward about 50cm and laterally about 20cm. Your left foot must be slightly on the left at 11 o'clock.

2. Bring up your arms at shoulder height.

**Start the exercise**

1. Stretch your right leg and bend your left leg.

2. Bring back your arms just behind your hips.

3. Stretch your left leg and bend your right leg.

4. Return your arms to the initial position at shoulder height.

5. Stretch your right leg and bend your left leg.

6. Bring back your arms just in front of your chest.

7. Stretch your left leg and bend your right leg.

8. Return your arms to the initial position at shoulder height.

Continue the sequence for 30 more times.

You can start with the first 4 movements until you feel you have them well stored in your mind and only after performing the entire sequence.

This exercise is very important also for the balance of your body to find the right position to receive the gravity force in a proper manner.

# The Movement Behind Taichi

As we have learned, Taichi is based on movements mainly with the tailbone, pelvis, legs, knees, arms, hands, and shoulders. The main mistake is to move your arms instead of your torso and one of the main difficulties is moving your hands in the right direction.

It is essential to learn how to do the movements correctly. Master Ping suggests 10 exercises that, if repeated several times, make the movements during Taichi more fluid and correct.

Before performing them, it is good to understand these four sequences:

1. Bend and extend the legs, then move the pelvis to the right and left. When there is a movement to the right, the knee of the right leg must bend and that of the left leg extends and vice versa, Then the pelvis moves to the right keeping the trunk still and well vertically. In each new pelvis movement to the right or left, it is important to first bend and extend the legs and then move the pelvis. Once the pelvis has been rotated in one direction, the next movement is that of the legs and must take place as soon as the hands cross on the vertical lateral line, then the pelvis and arms move.

2. Move the arms: The arms move together with the pelvis and continue the movement slightly up to the center line of the body and no further. Looking at the movements during Taichi, you may have the impression that the arms move beyond this line, but this is because the pelvis also moves.

3. Moving the hand: The hand moves with the pelvis and trunk and sometimes must undergo a rotation of 180 degrees. In principle (but not always) when the trunk goes to the right the palms of the hand are facing right and slightly down, when the trunk goes left and slightly down, when

the hands go up vertically or down the palms of the two hands are in the opposite direction.

4. Balance the shoulder: the shoulders should not be raised or lowered but remain still and well balanced with respect to the head.

To metabolize and make these movements your own, it is good to repeat the exercise many, many times on a regular basis for at least the first 60 days of practice.

I would therefore suggest repeating some of the following exercises every day, 14 times each.

## One hand

### Starting position

1. Move your left leg about 30cm on the left.
2. Put your left hand on your flank.
3. Bring your right hand with the palm down at the height of your right shoulder.

Exercise

## First circle

1. Bring your right hand down.
2. Stretch your right leg and bend your left knee, shift to the left your bust and follow the movement with the right hand until your right hand reaches the center line of your body.
3. Bring up your right hand with the palm up to the height of the left shoulder and turn it 180 degrees and stretch your left leg and bend your right knee and turn your head on the right.

4. Shift to the right your bust and follow the movement with the right hand with the palm to the right until your right hand is at the center line of your body.

Continue the sequence many times.

## Second circle

1. Starting position – see n.4 of the first circle.

2. Stretch your right leg and bend your left knee, shift to the left your bust and follow the movement with the right hand with the palm to the left until your right hand is at the center line of your body.

3. Bring down your right hand with the palm down to the height of the left hip, stretch your left leg and bend your right knee and turn your head on the right.

4. Shift to the right your bust and follow the movement with the right hand with the palm down until your right hand is at the center line of your body.

5. Rotate the palm of the right hand 180 degrees and bring your right hand up with the palm up to the initial position.

Continue the sequence many times.

## Third circle

### Starting position

1. Move your left leg about 30cm on the left.

2. Put your right hand on your flank.

3. Bring your left hand with the palm down at the height of your left shoulder.

**Exercise**

1. Bring your left hand down

2. Stretch your left leg and bend your right knee, shift to the right your bust and follow the movement with the left hand with the palm to the right until your left hand is at the center line of your body.

3. Bring up your left hand with the palm up to the height of the right shoulder and turn it 180 degrees and stretch your right leg and bend your right knee and turn your head to the left.

4. Shift to the left your bust and follow the movement with the left hand with the palm to the left until your left hand is at the center line of your body.

5. Continue the sequence many times.

## Fourth circle

1. Starting position – see n.4 of the third circle.

2. Stretch your left leg and bend your right knee, shift to the right your bust and follow the movement with the left hand with the palm to the right until your left hand is at the center line of your body.

3. Bring down your left hand with the palm down to the height of your right hip and stretch your right leg and bend your left knee and turn your head on the left.

4. Shift to the left your bust and follow the movement with the left hand with the palm down until when your left hand is at the center line of your body.

5. Rotate your left hand and bring it back with the palm up to the start position.

6. Continue the sequence many times.

## Two hands

### Fifth and sixth circles

**Starting position**

1. Move your left leg about 30cm on the left.

2. Bring your right hand with the palm forward, up to the right at shoulder height and your left hand with your palm down, down to the height of your left hip.

**Exercise**

Move both hands as in the first and third circle and as in the second and fourth circle.

## Seventh circle

**Starting position**

1. Move your right leg about 50cm behind and 20cm on the right with your feet at 3 o'clock.

2. Turn your bust on the right at 2 o'clock, raise your hands in front of the chest with the palm forward.

**Exercise**

1. Stretch your left leg and bend your right knee, shift to the right your bust and follow the movement with the hands until when your left hand reaches the center line of your body.

2. Bring down your hands with the palm down to the height of your right hip and stretch your right leg and bend your left knee and turn your head to the left.

3. Shift to the left your bust and follow the movement with both hands, with both palms down until your right hand is at the center line of your body.
4. Rotate both hands and bring them up.
5. Bring them back with the palm on the right to the starting position.
6. Continue the sequence many times.

## Eighth circle

### Starting position

1. Move your right leg about 50cm behind and 20cm on the right with your feet at 3 o'clock.
2. Turn your bust on the right at 2 o'clock, raise your hands in front of your chest with palms facing forward.

### Exercise

1. Stretch your right leg and bend your left knee, shift to the left your bust and follow the movement with your hands until right hand reaches the center line of your body.
2. Bring down your hands with the palm down to the height of your left hip and stretch your left leg and bend your right knee and turn your head on the right.
3. Shift to the right your bust and follow the movement with both hands with palm down, until your left hand is at the center line of your body.
4. Rotate both hands and raise them.
5. Bring them back with the palm on the left to the starting position.
6. Continue the sequence many times.

## Ninth and tenth circles

The same as seventh and eighth but as starting position move your left leg about 50cm behind and 20cm on the left with the feet at 9 o'clock.

# The force of gravity

Just after my eleventh day in China I had already changed my mindset. The main concept I have metabolized most quickly is that of the force of gravity. The idea is to let the force of gravity come from your head into your body and let it flow down freely without any blockage to the feet and then to receive it back up to your head.

Quite excited, I shared my experience with my friends Alvydas, Jyun and Mike. In the short discussions you can have on WhatsApp, this enthusiasm of mine in having understood and experienced on my body the sense of the force of gravity, was multiplied in hearing even more holistic and extraordinary statements on this topic.

Alvydas's wish for a "*wonderful experience on this new dimension*", has motivated me, if possible, even more, to experiment with this concept through an even greater commitment to putting my body in a position to do so.

Mike added that "*there are two functional premises regarding health: neutrality to gravity and cellular optimization*" (there is a third one that I can share if we may have once the chance to meet), I realized I was well on my way to reaching this state with the integration of EnergyUpbiotics (see description of the product in dedicated chapter at the end of this book) and the practice of the Taichi.

When I then found out from Jyun's words that even emotions are affected by the force of gravity my heart and mind lit up immensely – *Mi illumino d'immenso* to quote two epic verses by Ungaretti. In fact, Jyun states that "*The dynamic point of view regarding gravity emphasizes the subjective experience of gravitational forces as they relate to human beings. Rather than seeing gravity solely as a physical force that acts uniformly on all objects, this perspective highlights how individuals perceive and respond to gravity in various contexts. From this viewpoint, gravity is not just a constant force; it interacts with our physical bodies and consciousness in nuanced ways. For example, the sensation of weight can vary depending on our emotional state, activity level, and even our environment (e.g., feeling lighter when jumping or heavier during intense physical exertion). This subjective experience shapes our understanding of movement, balance, and stability. Moreover, the dynamic perspective considers how gravity influences our relationships with the world around us. It affects how we navigate spaces, interact with others, and even how we conceptualize our place in the universe. In essence, the dynamic point of view invites us to explore gravity not just as a scientific principle but as a lived experience that intertwines with our perceptions, emotions, and interactions, ultimately shaping our existence as human beings".*

# The puppet

When my father died, about ten years ago, I had sorted the objects I would keep at our holiday home in the Monti. There was not much left except for a few objects, perhaps no more than five. Two of these were puppets. I don't know why my father had bought them and always kept them in plain sight. Perhaps, in a quantum context of no space and no time, he had perceived the symbolism of these theatrical puppets in their logic of moving in a dynamic perfectly consistent with the force of gravity.

I like to share this anecdote to draw your attention to just how puppets move.

There is a piece of wood to which ropes are attached, which in turn supports the head, arms and legs.

I ask you to now close your eyes and imagine yourself as a puppet. Imagine your light head, which must not carry any weight and thought, imagine your arms raised in front of your chest moving dynamically on their own, imagine your legs swinging from the pelvis light.

Now, the puppet that you are, is placed on the ground and you feel your feet touch the ground decisively. You perceived a good feeling of belonging to the earth, but your head continues to be light, your arms free to swing. You feel the force of gravity descend from your head down to your feet without encountering any obstacles. You feel it strongly on your feet that you support you generously and are ready to give you back the strength you need at the right time.

Welcome to a dynamic body that accepts the force of gravity and uses it to our advantage.

I like to think that my father was able to turn into a puppet and finally found the tranquility he had never achieved.

# Running and meditation

In my understanding of the benefits of meditation, I immediately thought about how this practice could benefit running. I reiterate that the meditation in question is not the end of reaching a hypnotic state but is functional to help the consciousness to move the vital energy which in turn helps to move the body. It is about being able to focus your attention inside your body and to share it with the force of gravity. Meditation allows you to balance your bone structure to make it stronger as well as tendons and ligaments more elastic, it allows you to relax your body, your muscles.

I therefore wondered if this could also be put to the benefit of running and I think the answer is affirmative. In fact, it is the goal of both meditation and running to neutralize the force of gravity.

In meditation we try to stretch the back upwards and towards the pelvis, we try to make the body lighter, relax the muscles, put the weight on the feet. During meditation, the mind is focused on the body and on nothing else. Since the body has a larger memory than the mind, this habit manages to create an automatism that over time is then replicated automatically. And it is precisely on this aspect that meditation can help running. The gesture of running becomes more efficient if you can relax your body by taking full advantage of the force of gravity. Light shoulders, a relaxed neck, loose arms, flexible pelvis and stable legs allow the force of gravity to descend from the head to the feet with all its force that can then be exploited in the athletic gesture. If you can replicate the dynamics that are put in place in meditation during running, your body will be lighter and more efficient.

So, I like to think that I can introduce meditation sessions into the running training program. Two, three times a week, 30-minute sessions allow you to program your body so that it can memorize neutrality with respect to gravity.

Memory that the body can then exploit during the race. Initially, to promote this memorization process, during recovery and slow running sessions you can retrace the focus you have during meditation. Correct posture, relaxed shoulders and muscles, flexible pelvis, stable legs, upward stretching of the back.

Over time, the body autonomously implements this dynamic, allowing better performance.

# EnergyUpprobiotic

It has now been 4 months that I'm taking this unique product, and I can firmly say that I have been experimenting its benefits mainly on the digestion which for many years had been a real problem that decrease my quality of life. I can also safely say that my skin has become extremely soft.

I'm not the type of person who likes to promote products, and I only do it if I firmly believe in the product I propose. I had the chance to meet the person who created EnergyUpprobiotic and I have experienced his extraordinary generosity and desire to help others. Alydas is now a trusted friend of mine.

It is not just a probiotic; it is literally a *"lifestyle"* that also gives numerous benefits at cellular level.

Thanks to innovative cultivation technology, seven strains of probiotic bacteria reach the gut alive and active and are ready to improve Microbiome. This powerful formula combines special probiotic bacteria and Red Korean Ginseng to optimize intestinal function, enhance nutrient absorption, support a healthy gut, balance immunity and fuel your body's energy production, providing vitality throughout the day. This path leads to longevity.

## Red Korean Ginseng & Probiotics

Fermented Red Korean Ginseng and the patented probiotic blend work in synergy for exceptional bioavailability and efficacy. Red Korean Ginseng, safely used for over 4,500 years, is celebrated as the root of longevity and the elixir for the "five viscera." Thanks to fermentation and probiotic synergy, its extract is optimized for vitality, healthy gut and overall body support.

## Gut health boost

Most probiotics struggle to survive the harsh journey through the gastrointestinal tract. This innovative delivery system, reinforced with a silk fibroin coating, enhances bacterial viability and adhesion, fostering beneficial growth while preventing harmful colonization.

### Satisfaction

98% of users positively evaluated the taste and form of consumption. 85% of users felt the effects of Red Korean Ginseng and probiotics within the first week of use.

### Recommendations for use

Recommended to use as a dietary supplement:

- ✓ An exceptional form of use - "melting in your mouth"
- ✓ Excellent taste
- ✓ Once or twice a day after the meals
- ✓ Comfortable packages you can have with you everywhere

### What do consumers feel after 2-3 months of use:

- ✓ Balanced Mental Activity
- ✓ Improved blood circulation
- ✓ Return of youth
- ✓ Vitality
- ✓ Efficient immunity
- ✓ Improved Memory

You can melt the powder directly in your mouth or prepare a drink with 50ml of 40C water. Use it after your meal in the morning or at lunchtime.

### How to buy it

To get a 6% discount, you can buy through this link **EnergyUpbiotic.**

# Practice

My advice for those who want to start practicing QiGong or Taichi is to try to do a series of trial lessons with a master. From my experience, to understand if it could be a discipline to undertake, at least 25 hours of lessons are needed.

Once this "obstacle" has passed, you begin to enter the splendid dynamics of its movements and begin to perceive the benefits. In China, it is said that it takes 100 days of daily practice to fully enter this discipline. Once we have crossed this border, no one can stop us.

Taichi is a rather difficult discipline to learn correctly, and it is therefore important to find a qualified teacher who is able to transmit the theory by talking about warm-up, movements, breathing, meditation, the force of gravity. He must also dedicate time, propose and explain specific exercises to improve posture and movements. A Taichi practice without specific accompaniment will not be of much use because the movements will not be done correctly.

To get started, I highly recommend taking an intensive course of at least one week for at least 25 hours of practice.

In this book I don't feel like proposing a daily or weekly program, because everyone must find his own way. At dawn, during the morning, in the midday break, in the afternoon, at sunset, in the evening (not before sleeping), Qigong and Taichi can find their space. 30 minutes of repeated activity once, twice or three times a day is enough.

# B&B Cuore Alpino

Together with my wife Sara, we are the owners of the B&B Cuore Alpino that lends itself very well to retreats of various kinds, especially in disciplines such as yoga, meditation, etc., and certainly also in Taichi.

We have a very fragrant stone pine wood room suitable for lessons or simply to carry out the activity that in good weather can also be done in the beautiful garden that surrounds the property. The pure air that you breathe in this magical place in the Swiss Alps at 1000 meters above sea level allows Qi to circulate and integrate with the energy present in this unique place.

For those interested in carrying out their activity in our structure or those who would like to come and try a Qigong or Taichi lesson, you can contact us at this email address,
alloggioa5cuori@gmail.com.

Our magical Cuore Alpino can be seen at this site https://www.cuorealpino.ch/

# Conclusion

During my 30-day stay in China, I entered the wonderful world of Qigong in the 8 forms of Baduanjin and the 12 Yi Jin Jing, as well as the even more extraordinary world of Taichi in the 10 basic forms and, especially in the 18 forms of Chen Taichi. In total I learned 48 shapes for over 500 different movements.

I have completed about 100 hours of lessons, and I think I can safely say that this discipline has entered my soul and will affect my life, although I have learned maybe one percent of this beautiful art.

If you are reading this conclusion, it means that maybe I managed to attract your attention and I could not be happier.

Life has been very generous with me and continues to smile at me. In my first book "La disillusione dell'essere" – which you can find on Amazon and Kindle – I ask myself what happiness is and I do it in a very rational way. Perhaps precisely because I was unable to find a definitive answer, fate or vital energy led me to look for other ways. This experience is proof of this, and I am convinced that it will make my already splendid and fortunate life even more extraordinary.

I take up the wishes of my beautiful wife Sara received for this trip, and I also share it with you. A wish that magically turned into a revelation.

I wish you something serious: LIGHTNESS

Evviva la vita, evviva il Qi.

Avanti tutta.

Andrea

# About the Author

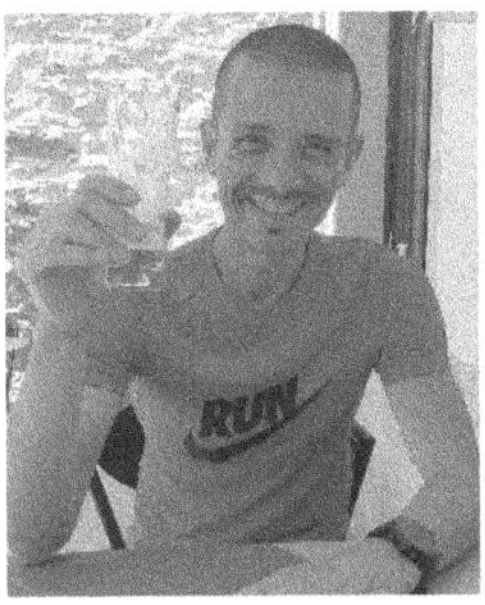

Andrea Laffranchini, with a degree in Economics and Human Resources, was born on 1. December 1966 in the Canton of Ticino in Switzerland, he is passionate about life. His motto "life is beautiful" is as simple as it is profound and suggests an intense path, sometimes suffered but in full evolution. On September 3, 1997, he had the extraordinary fortune to meet the woman of his life, Sara, and together they began a journey that was simply authentic, respectful, of listening and mutual help, of great understanding and infinite growing love.

A great lover of sport, Andrea Laffranchini has made it a lifestyle. He is a great fan of cross-country skiing, skiing touring and running. And it was in the latter, in his older age, that he achieved decent results as Swiss champion of the 800 meters, Swiss vice-champion of the 1500 meters, Ticino vice-champion of cross-country running.

Passionate about nature, in 2018 he followed a 60-day intensive course as a middle mountain guide.

Director of the Sports Authority of the City of Bellinzona and co-owner with his wife of the unique B&B Cuore Alpino in Olivone, a beautiful village in Italian-speaking Switzerland, he continues to cultivate his passion for "doing" through various projects both in the naturalistic and educational fields.

In 2024 he meets extraordinary people who mark the beginning of a new chapter oriented towards health at 360 degrees, especially in the sports field. People who stimulate him to a better understanding of the functioning of the human body and that led him to travel to China in March 2025 for an intensive course in Qigong and Taichi.

Experience that motivates him to write this book.

# Qigong & Taichi Certification

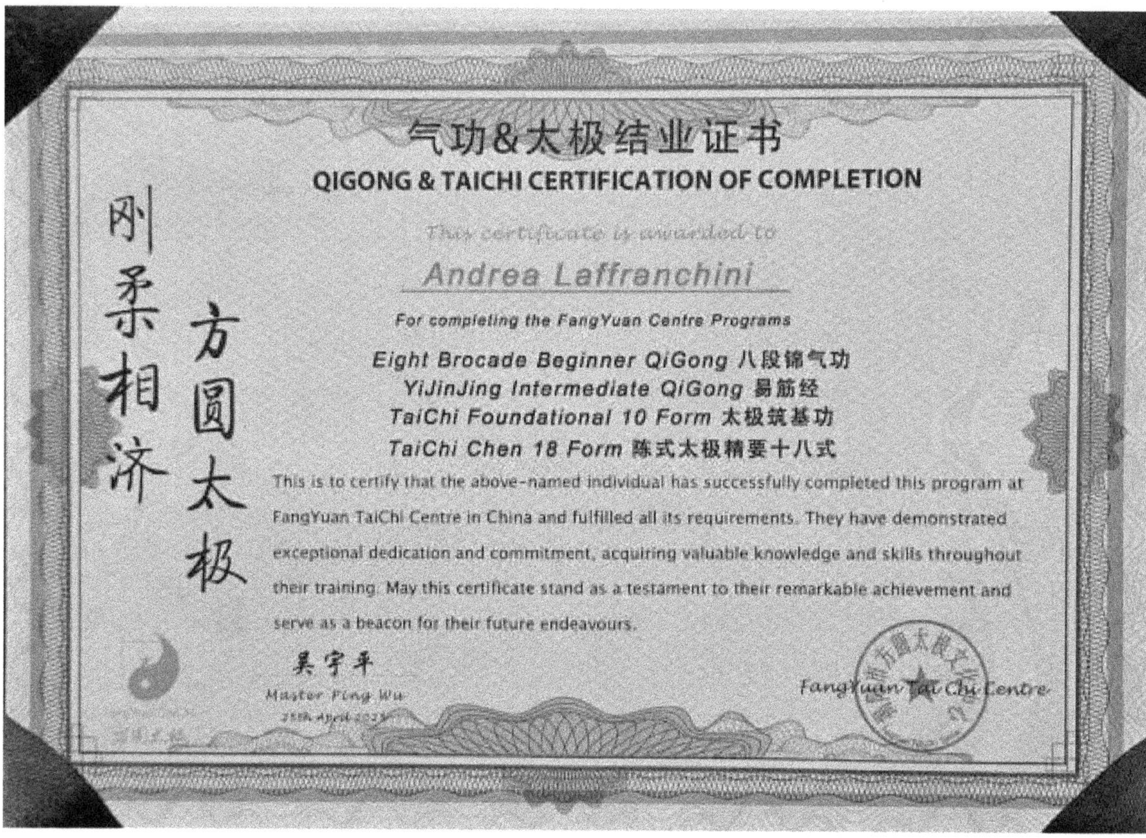

刚柔相济 方圆太极

气功&太极结业证书

QIGONG & TAICHI CERTIFICATION OF COMPLETION

This certificate is awarded to

Andrea Laffranchini

For completing the FangYuan Centre Programs

Eight Brocade Beginner QiGong 八段锦气功
YiJinJing Intermediate QiGong 易筋经
TaiChi Foundational 10 Form 太极筑基功
TaiChi Chen 18 Form 陈式太极精要十八式

This is to certify that the above-named individual has successfully completed this program at FangYuan TaiChi Centre in China and fulfilled all its requirements. They have demonstrated exceptional dedication and commitment, acquiring valuable knowledge and skills throughout their training. May this certificate stand as a testament to their remarkable achievement and serve as a beacon for their future endeavours.

吴宇平
Master Ping Wu

FangYuan Tai Chi Centre

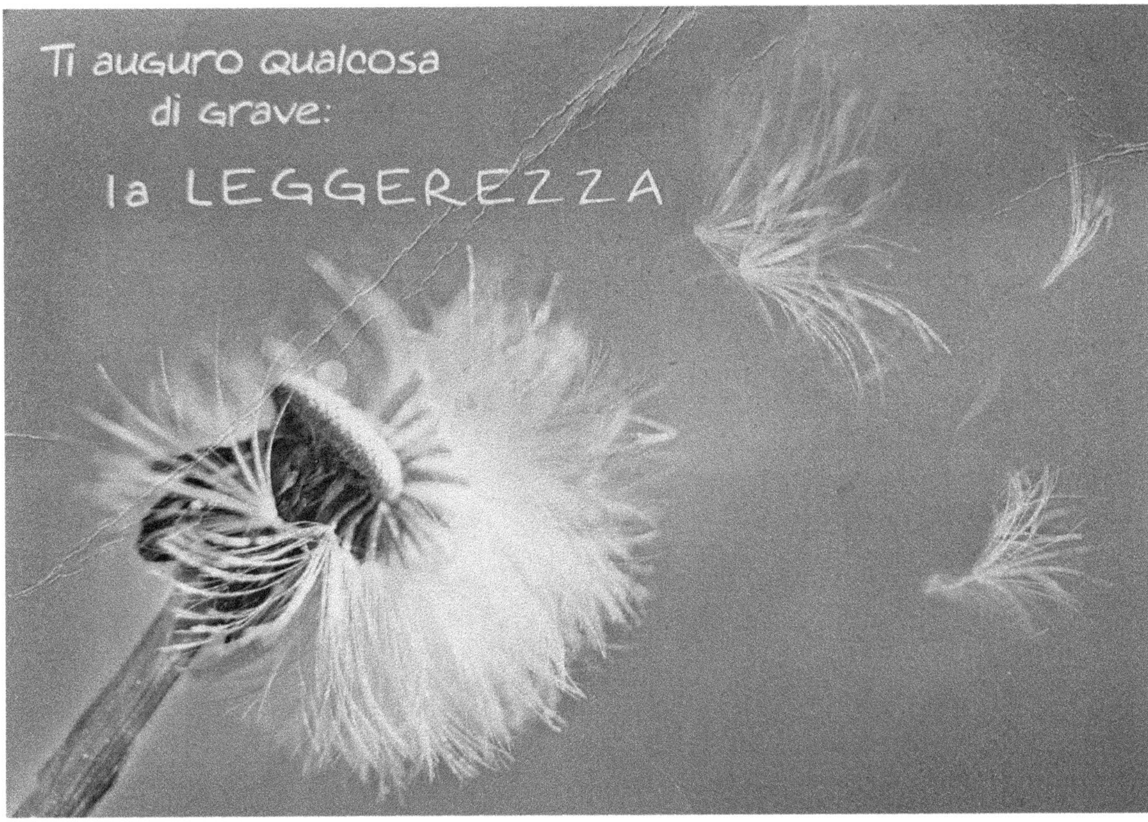


*If you don't believe there is a vital energy that circulates in our body and is part of something bigger, if you believe that you have a scientific mind, then this is the book for you.*

*Accept the force of gravity, in addition to being a personal story full of emotions, a journey of simple and deep connection with one's being, it is also a very rational account of the benefits of practicing Taichi.*

*In his story, the author manages to make the measurable coexist with the immeasurable, the circumscribed with the boundless: force of gravity with meditation, human body with energy, meridians with organs. In reading it, one does not have the opportunity or the temptation to question some concepts, because they simply and magically enter the mind.*

*Reading this book is like stepping into a dream. Once the cover is closed, you wake up and you have the impression that it is all so true. One has the impression of having entered a dimension of non-space and non-time. You want to start discovering this magical discipline.*

*Reading this book makes you understand how age is just a number and that everyone can start practicing this discipline and everyone can thus have the privilege of experiencing and living the vital energy that exists in us.*

*The force of gravity through Newton's theory of the apple suddenly and simply becomes an incredible truth that goes beyond the purely scientific one.*

www.ingramcontent.com/pod-product-compliance
Lightning Source LLC
Chambersburg PA
CBHW041748220926
51847CB00013B/144
* 9 7 8 9 6 9 7 3 9 2 1 0 0 *